Lean Muscle Diet For Beginners:

Healthy Weight Loss Nutrition, Exercises and Workouts For a Perfect Body

By

Valerie Alston

Table of Contents

Introduction 5

Chapter 1. Why Lean Muscle Diet? 6

Chapter 2. Lean Muscle Diet Principles 7

Chapter 3. Tips For Best Results 12

Chapter 4. Which Foods to Eat 14

Chapter 5. Avoid This Food 18

Chapter 6. Calorie Intake For Women 19

Chapter 7. Vegetarian Food Recipes 20

Chapter 8. Your Best Diet Plan 23

    Sample Plan 23

Chapter 9. How to Gain Lean Mass Through Weight Training 25

Chapter 10. Post-Workout Meals 29

    Some Recipes 29

Chapter 11. Pre-Workout Meal 32

Conclusion 34

Thank You Page 35

Lean Muscle Diet For Beginners: Healthy Weight Loss Nutrition, Exercises and Workouts For a Perfect Body

By Valerie Alston

© Copyright 2015 Valerie Alston

Reproduction or translation of any part of this work beyond that permitted by section 107 or 108 of the 1976 United States Copyright Act without permission of the copyright owner is unlawful. Requests for permission or further information should be addressed to the author.

This publication is designed to provide accurate and authoritative information in regard to the subject matter covered. This work is sold with the understanding that the publisher is not engaged in rendering legal, accounting, or other professional services. If legal advice or other expert assistance is required, the services of a competent professional person should be sought.

First Published, 2015

Printed in the United States of America

Introduction

A diet to make lean muscles requires being high in calories and revolving around good foods. The total calorie intake, protein and carbohydrate in your diet will define how much muscle you can add, rather than the specific foods which deserve a place in your eating plan. High protein foods, overall-grain carbohydrates and healthy fats work great for that particular diet.

Everyone wants to enhance lean mass, but most of the people don't like the opinion of gaining body fat, even as slight as a couple of pounds, which is one of the best mass-gaining meal plans.

Chapter 1. Why Lean Muscle Diet?

By eating less, frequent meals, you form a small insulin spike. On the other hand, by eating infrequent meals, you create large insulin spikes that will consequence of a crash that can build the body extra prone to fat storage. Anyone doesn't accept this. Most of the people
Want to gain higher lean mass and little fat as possible as possible.

Maintain stable insulin levels through the day and take frequent, smaller meals to retain your metabolism revving in addition to keep your body full with nutrients to give your muscles with what they want to grow. Include fat with your meals. When you consume fat with any meal, mainly one having carbohydrates, it will encapsulate these carbohydrates and create your body release insulin at a slower and steadier rate than eating carbohydrates only.

Chapter 2. Lean Muscle Diet Principles

This diet takes a lot of factors, according to a meal by meal basis. The most attention in these areas is: amount of calories consumed, insulin control, macronutrient composition and maintaining an alkaline state.

Eat Enough Calories

You will most likely eat more on this diet than any moment in your life, the major factor in this diet is calories in contrasted with calories out. This diet also provides the food selections as well as the package you require to aid fuel muscle development while caring fat expansion to an complete least.

Macronutrient Manipulation

Now it's time to discuss about the macronutrient manipulation. The main key to developing figure is to make sure you get the exact amount of calories and that those calories create lean mass, not fat. You must take the right kind of food at the exact time.

Moreover, it is essential to know that insulin sensitivity was lowest at the time of night and highest earlier during the day. By taking carbohydrates when you are most active such as of the day and less when you are being more inactive at the nighttime.

Controlling Insulin Levels

Eat at least 5-8 meals daily: Large meals generate an enormous insulin spike, which is the result of your body to store fat. On the other hand, small meals make smaller insulin spike that can cause less fat storage in addition to more fat loss. Do not skip a meal. Try to keep the motor revving. Consume fat with all meals, especially meals including carbohydrates. Never combine carbohydrates and protein only because this elicits the greatest insulin response. For example, one cup oatmeal holds a moderate insulin response, however, when you mixed oatmeal with chicken, you can get a great higher response. If you do mix these, be confirming to add a fat source just like almonds or avocados.

Maintaining an Alkaline State

It is so much essential to control the acidity of your meals. How can you control this? Why does it matter? PH level of your body's is slightly alkaline, according to the normal range of pH is 7.36 to 7.44. To uphold optimal health and results, you might try to maintain your body in an alkaline state throughout the diet. An imbalanced diet with high in acidic foods creates your body more acidic. This can empty the body of alkaline minerals like sodium, potassium, magnesium, and calcium, and also making people prone to chronic and degenerative illnesses and possibly disrupting nutrient absorption.

For instance, when you take a meal just like Oatmeal and egg whites, you are consuming a very acidic meal. On the other hand, when you keep raisins as well as almonds in your Oatmeal and have several steamed vegetables with it, you are decreasing the acidity of that meal significantly.

Smart Growth

Building muscle needs to be increased in calories; specifically, to gain weight, it is so much essential to consume more calories than you can burn every day. But if you eat too much and reach overboard, you will start the fat-storing process. So you must eat just adequate to facilitate the muscle-building process, but not too much that you will increase fat along with it.

You can get a way for controlling the portion sizes at mealtime. For most meals, you must take forty to sixty grams of protein and forty to eighty grams of starchy carbs, according to your size; bigger guys reaching more than, 225 pounds will shoot for the higher end. Dietary fat must be as low as possible, with the exception of healthy fats, which can extend to 5-10 grams per meal.

Meal Strategy

Eat 4-6 meals daily, and every meal must have carbs, protein, and some fat. Perfectly each meal contains equal in calories, but since it is normally you will do lunches and dinners for pleasure, the subsequent plan is most recommended.

Consume around 35% proteins, about 50% carbs, and about 15% fat.

How the Lean Mass Diet Works

This diet is very easy to follow. Provide a larger variety of popular, nutrient compact foods that are appropriately measured out to one serving.

These foods are also categorized in the subsequent manner:

1) Carbohydrate
2) Protein
3) Fats
4) Fruits
5) Vegetables
6) Milk

Every meal recommends a definite number of servings from the directly above categories based on your Dietary desires for your specific goals. Now an example can clear this. Meal one may recommend the subsequent:

a) 1 serving milk category
b) 1 serving fruit category
c) 3 servings carbohydrate category
d) 2 servings protein category
e) 2 servings fat category

Chapter 3. Tips For Best Results

This diet plan is completed with some fresh, clean foods that are as natural as possible. If you maintain some simple principles, you will shed fat so fast.

Try to take at least one gram of protein for each pound of bodyweight, every day. If you feel your protein consumption is as low as on a restricted diet of calorie, you will lose lots of muscle in addition to some fat you're fortunate enough to shed. High protein consumption should help you protect lean mass during dieting. You must select lean first-class proteins just like poultry, thin red meat, egg whites as well as protein supplements. This diet, which delivered here includes closer to 230- 240 g of protein per day, well for a male considering nearly 220-250 pounds. Increase your protein just only if you're very hungry or you're weightier than 250 pounds and want to add some extra food during the day. Besides, if you're less than 180 pounds, cut out at least 3 ounces of meat from chicken daily from the diet.

When you try to lose some weight, keep your carbohydrates low to moderate. Besides, on a very short day you will have nearby 100 g of carbs. On the other hand, a modest day you will also have carbs of about 150g. Rotate little and modest days so as to retain the energy or power high and give a variation of step. Decent, fresh, healthy fiber-rich carbs contain oats, sweet potatoes, brown rice and whole ounce bread.

Drink no less than a 3litres of water daily. Drink water and lots of it because water is a key in absolutely all parts of fitness and nutrition. It will keep you healthy as well as hydrated. It also acts as a key in burning of fat. Water would be your main beverage during dieting. Besides this, drinking lots of calorie-free water can truly make you feel complete meaning that you're less likely to start snacking. Although many depend on diet sodas, and other low-calorie sugared drinks, moreover, plain old water is actually your best bet.

Chapter 4. Which Foods to Eat

It is an important question- which foods you can take at the time of lean dieting? Some natural whole grain as well as starchy carbs you can take at the time of dieting such as brown rice, sweet potatoes, white potatoes, beans, whole wheat bread, whole wheat pasta and yams. All of this natural starchy carbs actually aid weight loss owing to their high fiber content and are necessary for encouraging fat loss in addition to the growth of lean muscle.

You must take some lean proteins from egg whites, salmon, lean Ground Turkey, chicken breast, turkey breast and casein protein. All of these foods contain high proteins that are so much essential at the time of dieting.

You must eat lots of vegetables daily. Vegetables keep your body fit and make your skin so much gloomy. In this reason everyone keeps several vegetables at the mealtime. During diet, you can eat a lot of broccoli, Onions, Tomatoes, Cucumbers, Salad greens, Zucchini as well as Mushrooms.

Some fruits such as Apples, Strawberries, Grapes, Blueberries, Bananas, Pineapple, Oranges and Grapefruit must keep in your meal. When you try to diet, you must take lots of fruits and vegetables. Both fruits and vegetables are so much essential food for dieting. Everyone can eat fruits as much as he or she wants.

Brown rice

Brown rice might not taste fairly as well as white rice, but the brown stuff is very much healthier. Moreover, it's a very slow digesting whole grain that will give you with long-lasting energy for the period of your workouts. It is also recognized as boost your growth hormone levels, which are vital for encouraging fat loss and strength gains.

Sweet potatoes

Though Sweet potatoes are filled with carbs, they are great for gaining lean muscle. The carbs, which contained in sweet potatoes, keep your glucose stable, a main element in burning fat as well as preserving muscle. They are an exceptional carb that actually helps weight loss, but they have really retained you fuller for longer than many other starchy vegetables.

Eggs

Eggs are your best friend while it comes to increasing lean muscle growth as well as strength gains. Eggs contain the perfect protein, but this also contains some cholesterol in the yolk and assists at the platform for steroid hormones which is also a contributing factor. Eggs are also known as a serious muscle building food.

Lentils

Lentils would be your secret mass building weapon. They are also very cheap and have an extensive shelf-life. They cook up quickly just like in 10 minutes and One cup of cooked lentils holds nearly eighteen grams of protein and about forty grams of very slow digesting quality carbohydrates. The cooked lentils can be mixed in with brown rice, a salad or can be eaten as a standalone side dish.

Apples

Apples assist to prevent muscle fatigue and increase muscle strength owing to the specific polyphenols that they hold. Some recent research has also suggested that they speed up the fat burning process, and making them a perfect pre-workout snack.

Chapter 5. Avoid This Food

Some foods must not eat during the lean muscle diet. Avoid alcohol, sugar and some processed foods. Never take alcohol at the time of diet. It is so much harmful for you. Try to avoid some soft drinks because they contain a lot of sugar. Keep limit your consumption of sugar. Taking in simple sugars before training does fill liver glycogen stores as well as muscle, on the other hand too much sugar devoured at other times of the day that will be stored up as fat. Obviously we all want to satisfy our sweet tooth sometimes, occasionally a doughnut fair hit the spot, then moderation is key, so controlling your intake of sugar to fresh fruit is advised greatest of the time. Try to replace coffee or tea, sugary drinks with water with no added sugar obviously.

The foods to decrease in this type would be sugar, which contains candy, cakes, pies, etc. But it also comprises fruit. So must keep a limit of consumption of sugar. Sugar increases unnecessary fat.

Chapter 6. Calorie Intake For Women

If you weigh 150lbs and are just only eating 1,200 calories, you are not eating sufficient. That doesn't mean disruption the donut that means enlarging your protein consumption to start. A very common guide for calorie intake is at your body weight times 10-12. Example: 150lbs x 10 = 1500 cal.

You may be considering this is much food, but it is not sufficient for you. So, increase Your Protein and never Fear about Fat. You can eat Beef, chicken, turkey, fish, etc. Most of the women only take lean meat only which isn't necessary. Enlarged protein helps keep the lean mass you already have. You want to retain this, as it improves your metabolism. Adding a little more lean mass is generally a good thing. If you take 40% of protein daily, you will see the great result.

Chapter 7. Vegetarian Food Recipes

Low-Fat, High-Protein Vegetarian Salad

This lovely, delicious dish contains almost 40g of protein without any meat! This vegetarian food contains high protein.

Ingredients:

You need six cups Shredded Lettuce, one cup Diced Orange Pepper, four large Egg Whites, chopped, half cup Tomato, chopped, one cup textured vegetable protein, two third cup Cooked Corn, half cup Low-Sodium Black Beans, and one forth cup barbecue sauce of choice.

How to do:

At first Cook textured vegetable protein according to package directions. Then combine textured vegetable protein with BBQ sauce. Then you add lettuce as well as veggies to salad bowl. Then top with textured vegetable protein. Top with salad dressing of choice. Then you can serve it.

Lentil Beans Soup

This vegetarian recipe might sound difficult, but if you keep all the ingredients, it's just simple to make.

Ingredients:

You need two tablespoons butter, one cup red lentils; one onion , chopped, two garlic cloves, crushed, half teaspoon turmeric, one teaspoon gram masala, 1/4 cups coconut milk, one teaspoon cumin, half cups vegetable stock, two teaspoons lemon juice, one forth teaspoon chili powder, one forth pounds preserved, sliced tomatoes. You can take salt and pepper to taste.

Cooking Instructions:

At first liquefy the butter in a pan and then put the onion and garlic in only for two minutes while rousing, then also must add the flavors and spices. Put in all tomatoes, lemon juice, red lentils, coconut milk, vegetable stock, and take to a boil. Decrease the warmth and seethe for twenty five to thirty minutes until the lentils are fully boiled. Then prepare to eat! It may hard to find, but it's really pretty easy. You don't want every ingredient, for it to still be good and it tastes so much delicious. You can add more coconut milk for a spicy taste.

Breakfast Drink

You can make a delicious breakfast drink with banana, almonds, yogurt etc.

Ingredients:

One fresh medium size banana, one cup plain yogurt, one hundred ml cold drinking water, one ounce ground almonds, one scoop protein powder and one cup raw oats

Cooking Instructions:

First, take all elements into a blender to blend, and then blend until it will be flat. Add drinking water if you like a feebler mixture. Then you can take it in a glass to drink.

Chapter 8. Your Best Diet Plan

Those who need to get ripped must have precise muscles as well as low amount of body fat. Have more fat to lose? Then you want to cut the calories. Remember, 1 pound is 3,500 calories. If you will decrease your daily consumption by 500 calories you will be unable to find 1 pound a week. If you want to enjoy yourself healthier, leaner and want to get ripped and control calories, you will consume an extensive selection of low calorie density as well as high mass foods.

Now here is a list of the greatest foods to eat. You must include them in your diet plan.

Sample Plan

In Breakfast you can take 4 egg whites, 2 whole eggs. Eggs, which are well known as a universal bodybuilding staple, provide easy-to-digest protein and kick-start muscle growth. Kashi Go Lean Cereal provides energy-rich complex carbohydrates.

When you want to Snack, you can eat 1 scoop whey protein and one tbsp. Peanut butter. If you want to consume more, you will take one medium size banana. Besides, bananas hold both fructose and potassium, which reduce muscle breakdown in the body and support the glycogen formation in the muscles as well as liver.

In Lunch you eat 2 slices of entire-wheat bread. Then you take again a can of white tuna with one tablespoon mayonnaise.

At Snack time you can eat 3 hard-boiled eggs with ¼ cup oatmeal. Then you can consume 10 oz. fresh spinach, and 2 tbsp. olive oil.

When you want to consume Dinner, you can consume only 10 oz. green beans, with 1 cup brown rice and 9 oz. Tilapia.

In Night-time snack, you can eat just only one scoop casein protein. It is not compulsory. If you need, you will take this night time snack.

Chapter 9. How to Gain Lean Mass Through Weight Training

Many of those who take weight training wish to know how they can create lean muscle mass so quickly. For this reason, you must learn the secrets behind weight training. So, you find the right way for building your muscle; otherwise, you are wasting time.

At first, you have to identify everything that is essential to the weight training program. Besides, you must identify about which exercises would be done on which days, and also know about how many reps to be done each set. Moreover, you have to plan about your mealtime for the day, and you must know how much calories that you eat every day. You must follow all basics for making lean muscle mass.

Compound Multi-Jointed Exercises

These compound multi-jointed exercises work on a large number of muscle groups than regular exercises. If you really want to attain big muscles rapidly, then you must maintain these exercises.

The following are specific of these exercises that can help in making lean muscle mass rapidly. You can also get some information on which muscle groups these compound multi-jointed exercises work.

- Squats (lower back and legs)

- Barbell rows and pull-ups (biceps)

- Overhead press (triceps and shoulders)

- Deadlifts (shoulders, back and legs)

- Bench press (triceps, shoulders and chest)

- Bar dips (arms, chest and shoulders)

Pull-ups and Barbell Rows Importance

Barbell rows and pull-ups are one of the greatest exercises that assist you to gain lean muscle quickly. Hence, make assured that you include these into your workout routine.

Heavy Weight Lifting

Lift heavy weights are essential for achieving lean muscle mass rapidly. It is as easy as that. You must not be worried about what others are lifting at your gymnasium. Just concentrate on your weight lifting and see your progress. Moreover, make sure that you should not be too weighty that they can injure you.

When you use the exact form and are able to perform 8 to 12 reps with every weight, then you understand that the weight is just right, perfect, abundant to challenge your body; if you aren't perform to do 7 reps, then you think that it is much heavier; and if you are able to execute more than 12 reps, at that moment, you understand that it is too little for your body. However, if you want to gain lean muscle, execute 7 to 12 reps to provide you the largest pains. Instead, if you want to increase the strength, then attempt doing 1 to 6 reps.

If you truly want to achieve lean muscle fast, then you must realize that long training sessions do not work perfectly! For best results, you have to make assured that the weight training session is less than an hour. Furthermore, you do not have to train every day. Three days in a week are enough. You can follow this mentioned time-table or any similar one. On Monday, biceps, back and arms, then Tuesday you take some break again Wednesday will be the legs, then the Thursday you must take a break further Friday will be triceps, shoulders and chest and then the Saturday and Sunday take a break.

The key to effective weight training for making lean muscle mass is planned workouts with sufficient rest and proper diet plan.

Chapter 10. Post-Workout Meals

Many of those who want to begin the muscle building process should recognize the process needs a quick dose of the exact carbohydrates and protein. Besides, you cannot always be dependent on rice, chicken as well as plain protein shakes. You can also choose an extensive variety of nutrient-dense foods. You try these excellent post-workout meals for getting the best result.

Some Recipes

Protein pancakes

Ingredients:

You need ½ cup cottage cheese, 4 egg whites, ½ teaspoon pure vanilla extract, ½ cup rolled oats, 1/8 teaspoon baking powder.

How to do:

Mix all elements. You must Cook on medium to low temperature until it bubbles, then and there flip and cool. Then this high protein pancakes with banana.

Important:

Persons who wish to get torn must take class post-workout nutrition. This is vital if you want to increase and quick gains. To improve your training outcomes faster, interchange glycogen as well as amino acids vanished during workout of the plan.

Tuna and Crackers

Elements:

You need half cup whole grain crackers, a can of yellow fin tuna

Procedure:

Combine the elements. For getting nice flavor, then take a dab of virgin oil, then pickles, mustard and pepper, cut up.

Large-Protein, Oats On-the-Go

Elements:

You need one or two scoops of whey protein powder, half cup of bowled oats, half cup of delicious fruit, and then you must dry or ice-covered slivered almonds.

Procedure:

Combine the ingredients. Then you can add a half cup of skim milk and then let it sit whole night in the refrigerator. Then you must add more nice flavors add cinnamon.

Chapter 11. Pre-Workout Meal

It is needed to take a pre workout mealtime at least 2 hours before you start your training. You can take 2 tablespoon of Peanut Butter and 2 revelations of Power Whey Protein

Peanut Butter

Peanut butter greatly tastes to add to snacks as like rice cakes, whole grain toast and as well to fruits such as apples and bananas. It is also a natural source of healthy carbohydrates, protein as well as fat. It also contains all the nutritional benefits. Besides, it can be intake at any time in the day, but adding a few to your pre-workout snack can give you with a source of long lasting energy.

What is Impact of the Whey Protein?

It has twenty grams of protein per serving. Whey protein has a wide-ranging amino acid profile providing all the vital amino acids (EAA's) and holds over 2g of Lucien each serving. Finest quality product whey protein offers an excellent value for currency and unbelievable flavor, appear no further. This high protein consumption will contribute to the growth as well as maintenance of lean muscle mass. This is an excellent choice which supports a wide variety of training goals.

Conclusion

The Lean Muscle Diet is very simple and solves the sustainability problem while providing immediate results. This diet provides a very simple, merely sustainable body transformation plan that any person can use. This diet helps you to gain weight loss using an easy, simple approach. You eat and train as if you at present have the body you want. You remain all the time in maintenance mode; you do not go off the diet because you do not go on a diet that expresses you what you can eat and can't eat!

Thank You Page

I want to personally thank you for reading my book. I hope you found information in this book useful and I would be very grateful if you could leave your honest review about this book. I certainly want to thank you in advance for doing this.

If you have the time, you can check my other books too.

www.ingramcontent.com/pod-product-compliance
Lightning Source LLC
LaVergne TN
LVHW021744060526
838200LV00052B/3470